MY BODY AND ME

My Healthy Bones

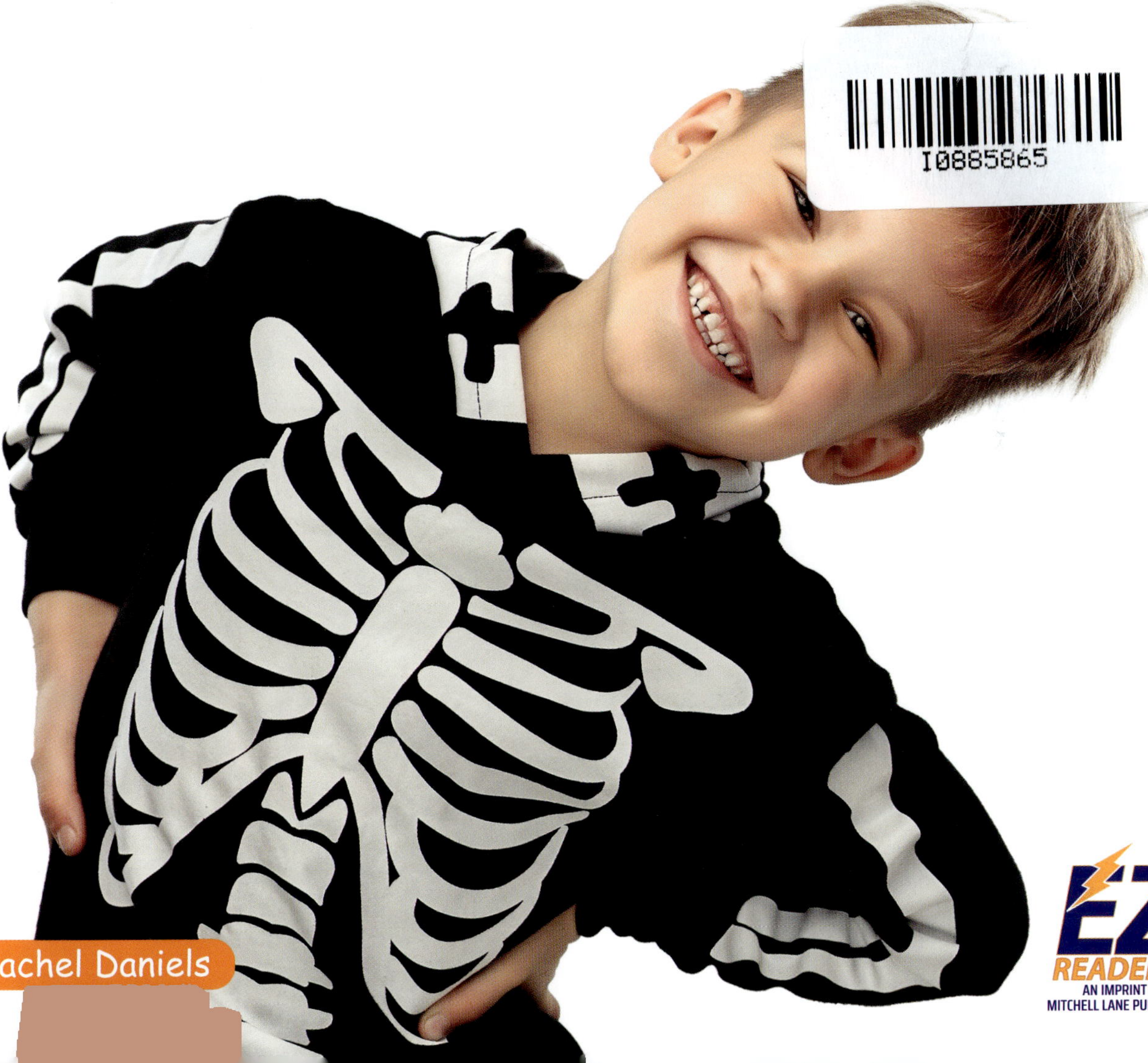

Rachel Daniels

EZ READERS
AN IMPRINT OF
MITCHELL LANE PUBLISHERS

CREATING YOUNG NONFICTION READERS

EZ Readers offer nonfiction for beginning readers in PreK through first grade, using simple language, clear illustrations, and engaging facts to build vocabulary and confidence.

TIPS FOR READING NONFICTION WITH BEGINNING READERS

Talk about Nonfiction

Begin by explaining that nonfiction books give us information that is true. The book will be organized around a specific topic or idea, and we may learn new facts through reading.

Look at the Parts

Most nonfiction books have helpful features. Our *EZ Readers* include color photographs and graphic aids, a table of contents, a glossary, and an index. Share the purpose of these features with your reader.

Color Photos and Graphic Aids

A lot of information can be found by "reading" photos, charts, maps, and other graphic aids found within nonfiction texts. Help your reader learn more about the different ways information can be displayed.

Table of Contents

Located at the front of the book, this list shows the big ideas within the text and the page numbers where they can be found.

Glossary

Located at the back of the book, the glossary defines key words and phrases that are related to the topic. These words and phrases can be found in the text in colored type.

Index

Located at the back of the book, an index is an alphabetical list of topics and the page numbers where they can be found.

With a little help and guidance about reading nonfiction, you can feel good about introducing a young reader to the world of *EZ Readers* nonfiction books.

EZ Readers is an imprint of:

Mitchell Lane
PUBLISHERS

2001 SW 31st Avenue
Hallandale, FL 33009
mitchelllanepub.com

First Edition, 2026.

Author: Rachel Daniels
Editor: Morgan Brody

ISBN 979-8-89260-827-5 (library binding)
ISBN 979-8-90145-033-8 (paperback)
ISBN 979-8-89260-832-9 (ebook)

LC record available at https://lccn.loc.gov/2025950886

Photo credits: Shutterstock, Alex Konon, cover, 1, 2, 3, 5, 6, 14, 17, 18, 21; Shutterstock, yusuf_demirci, cover, 1; iStock, dolgachov, cover, 1; Shutterstock, Sudowoodo, 3, 5, 7, 20; Shutterstock, CandyRetriever, 4, 22; Shutterstock, Marcin Balcerzak, 7, 22; Shutterstock, Creativa Images, 8; Shutterstock, FamVeld, 10–11; Shutterstock, sandsun, 12–13; Shutterstock, myboys.me, 15, 22; Shutterstock, Sergey Novikov, 16, 22; Shutterstock, kornnphoto, 19, 22; Shutterstock, Elena Chevalier, 20; iStock, Deagreez, 22; Shutterstock, NMK-Studio 22

Table of Contents

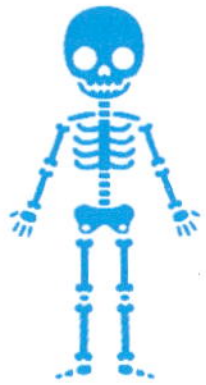

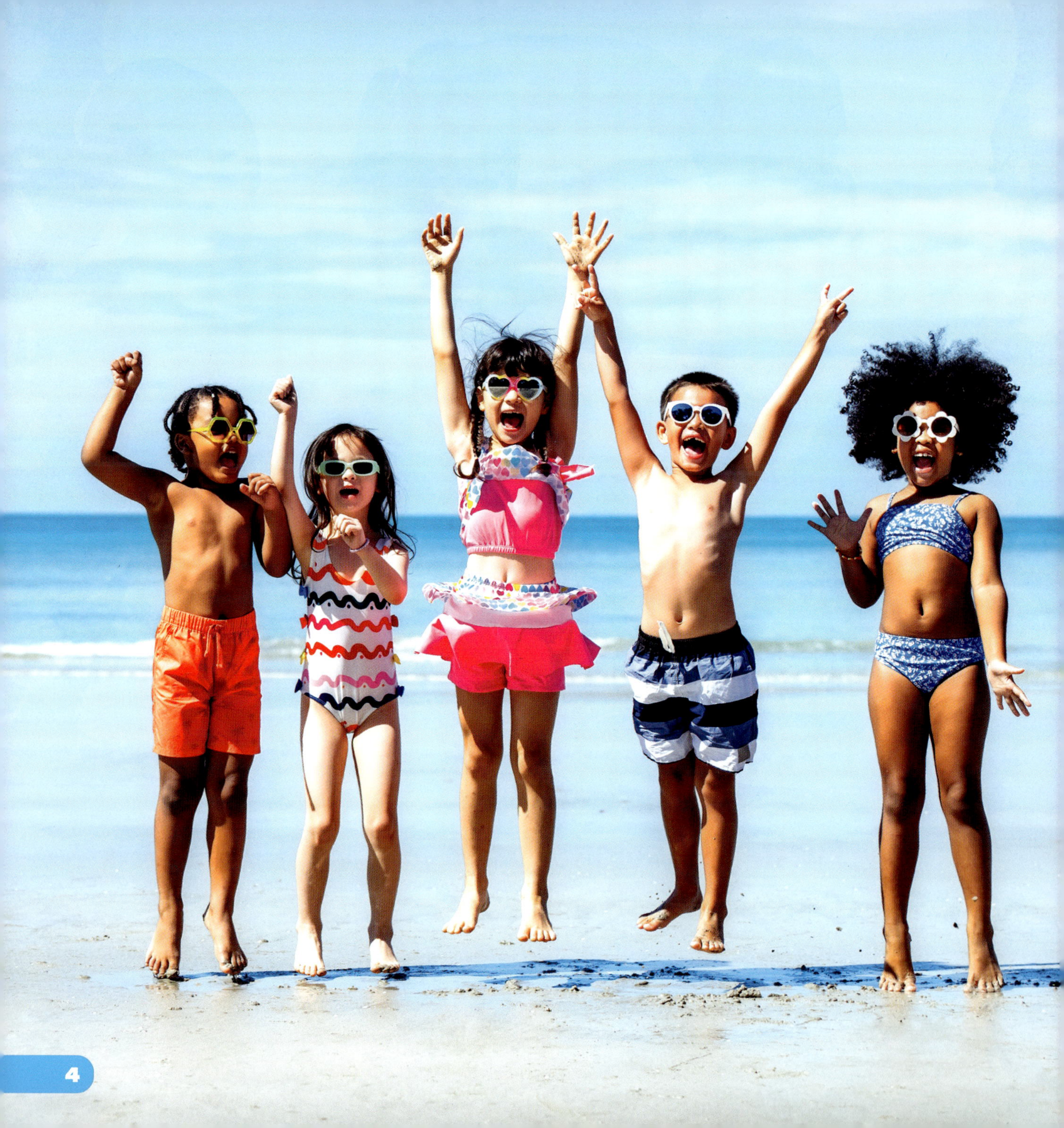

Strong Bones

Bones help me stand tall.
They help me run fast.
My bones make me **strong**.

BONE FACT!

Babies have more bones than grown-ups!

Inside My Body

Bones are under my skin.
They give my body **shape**.
Without bones, I'd be floppy!

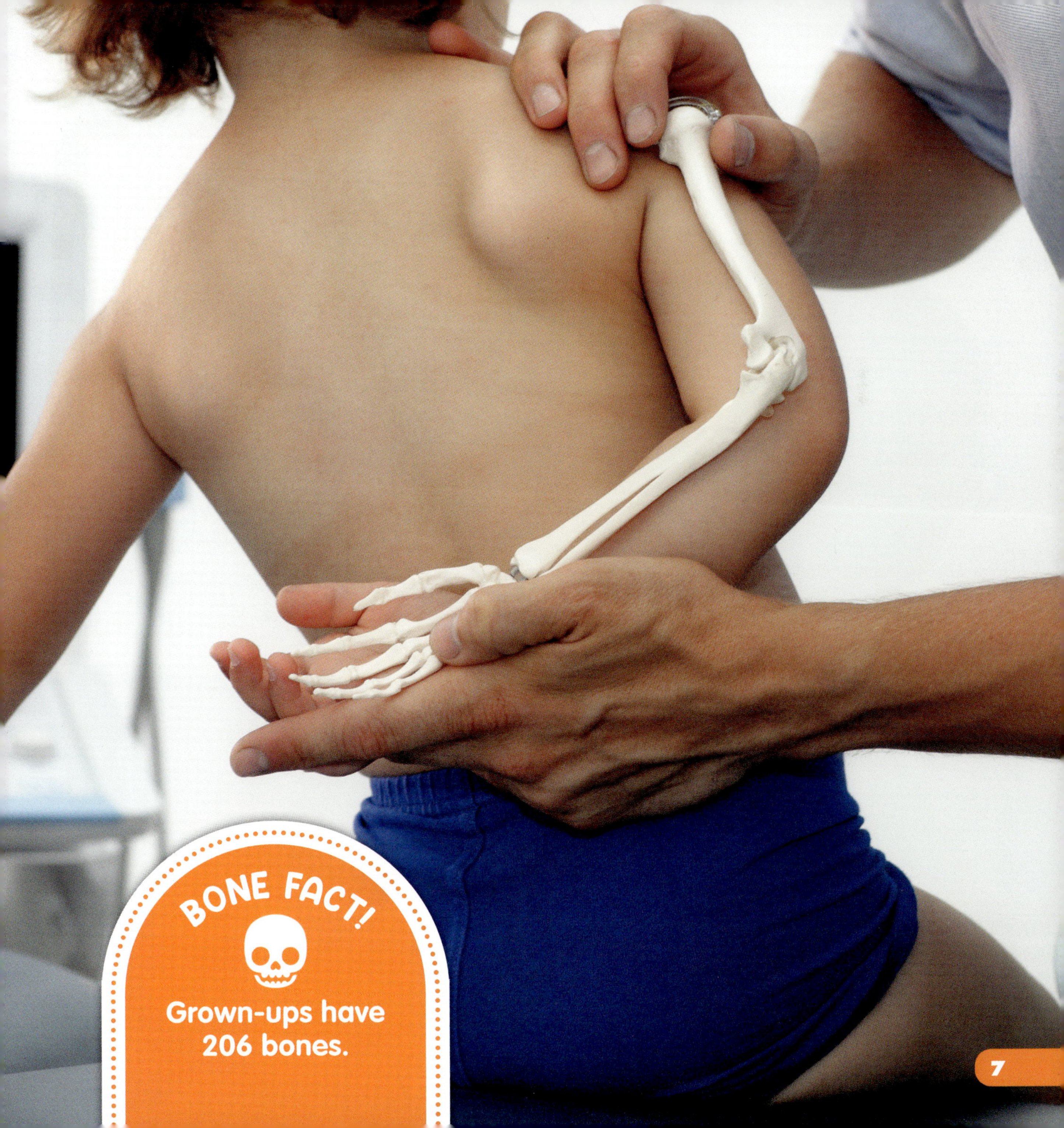

BONE FACT!

Grown-ups have 206 bones.

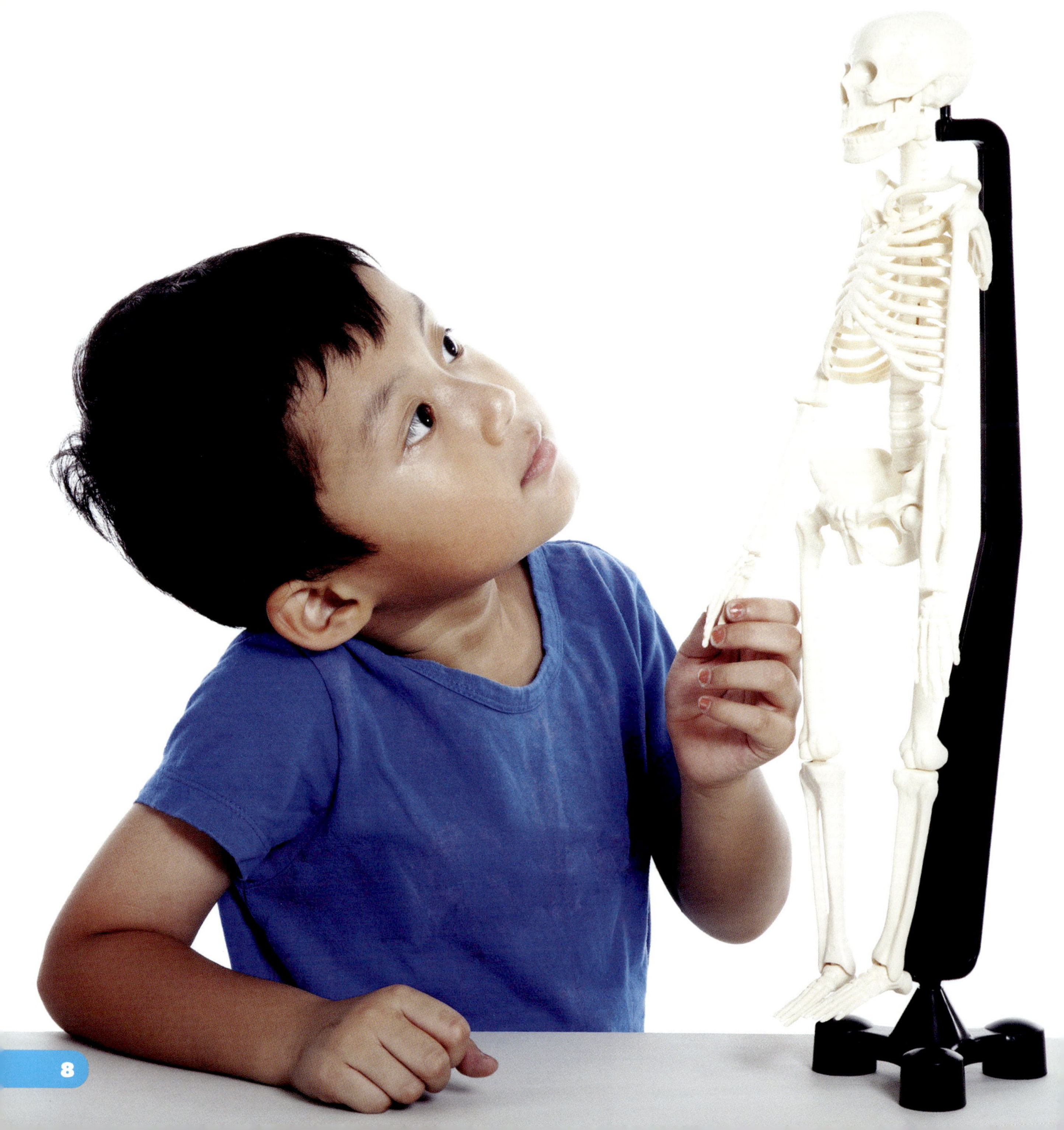

Bones are in my head.

Bones are in my toes.

Bones are everywhere!

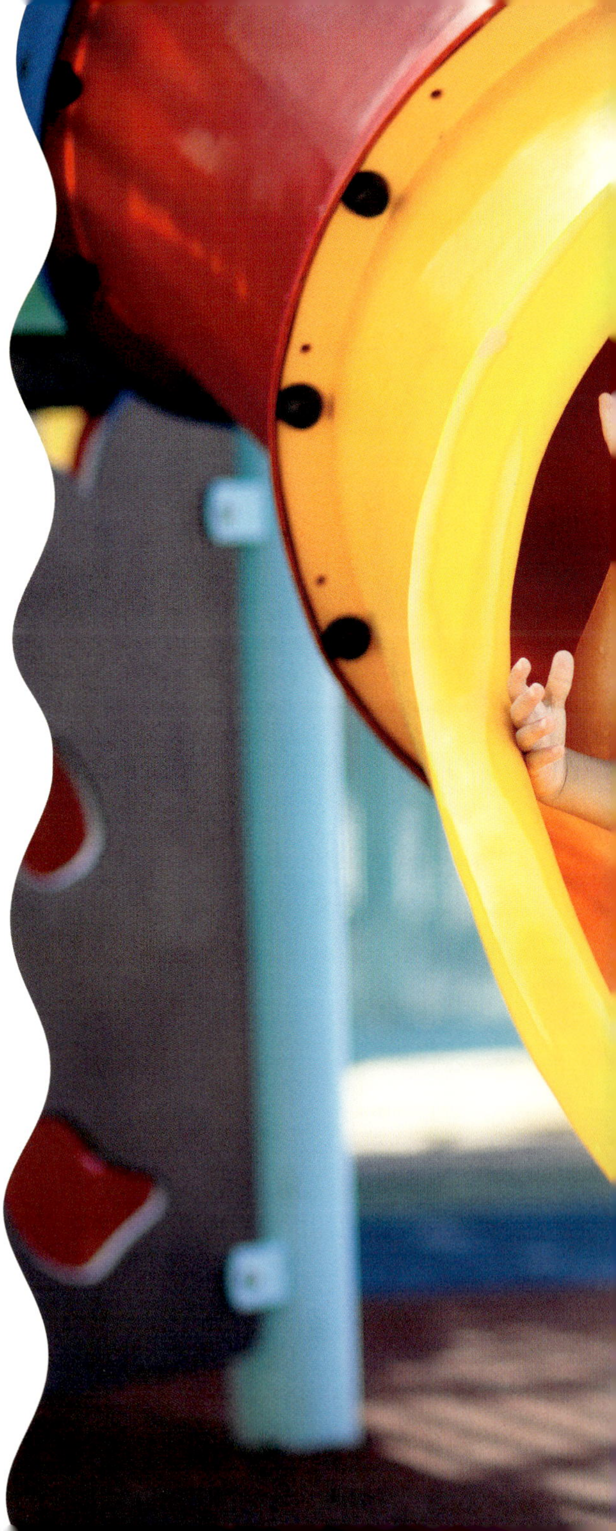

Bones bend at **joints**.

Knees move.

Elbows move.

Joints help me play!

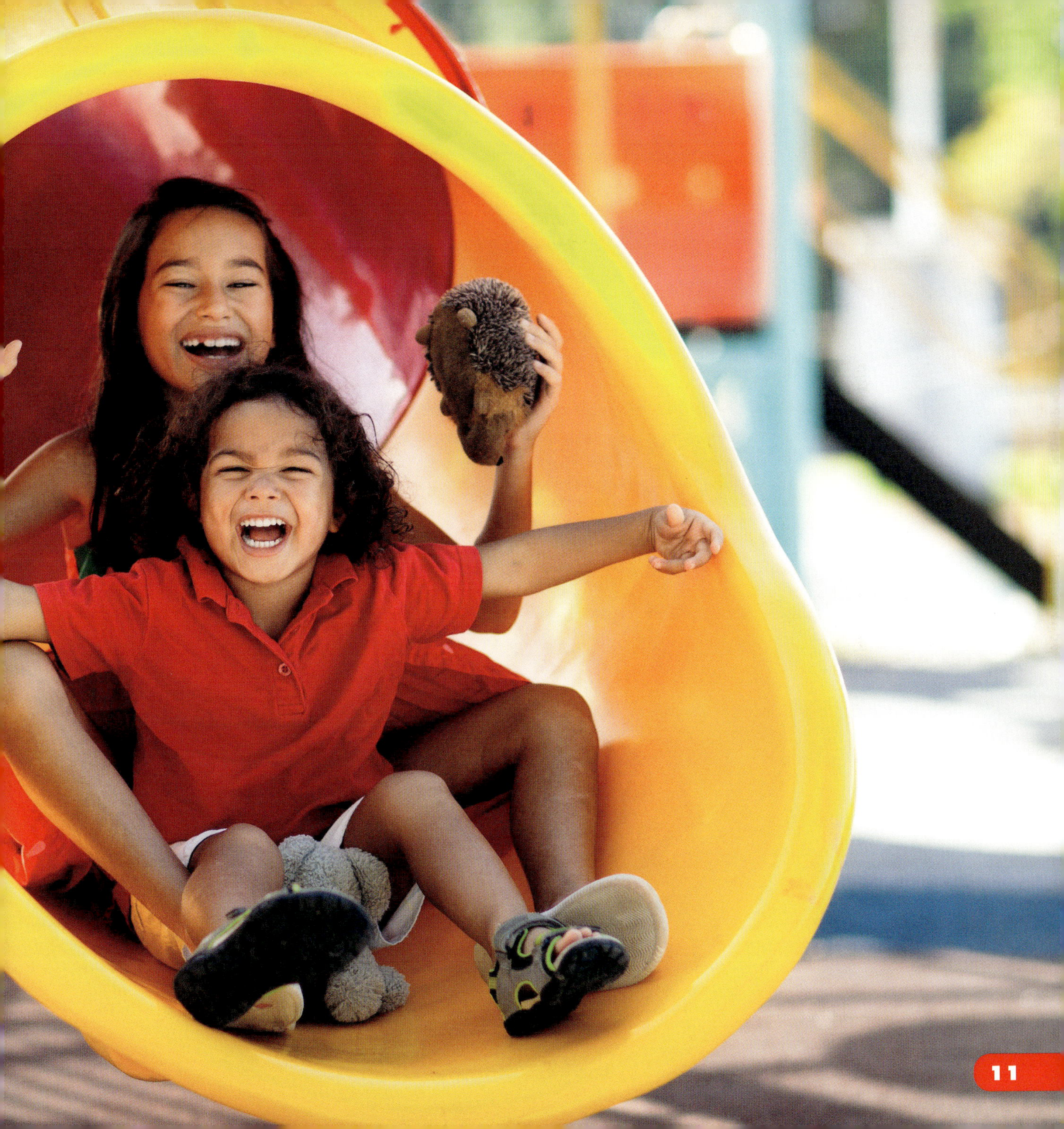

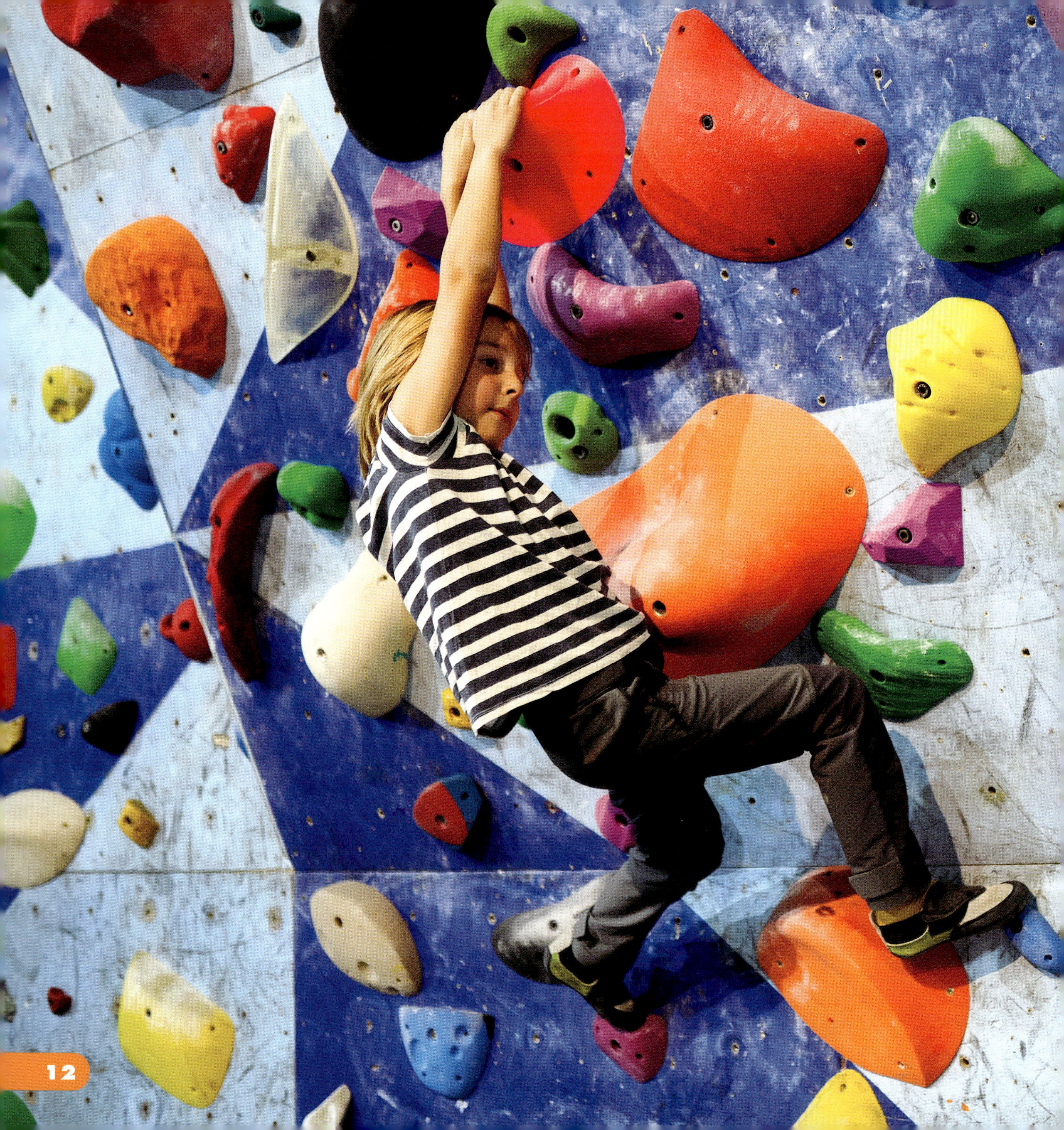

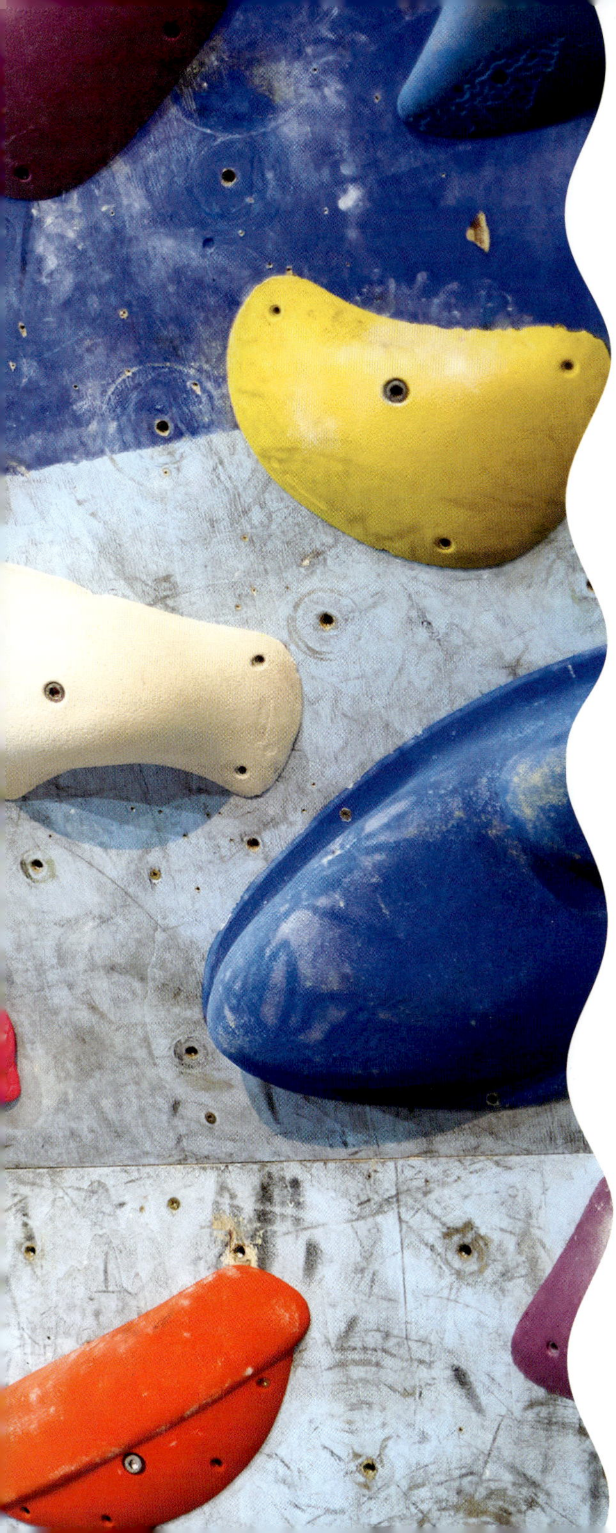

Bones and **muscles**
work together.

They help me lift.

They help me climb.

They help me run!

Food for Bones

Milk helps bones.

Cheese helps bones.

Greens help bones too.

Good food makes
bones strong.

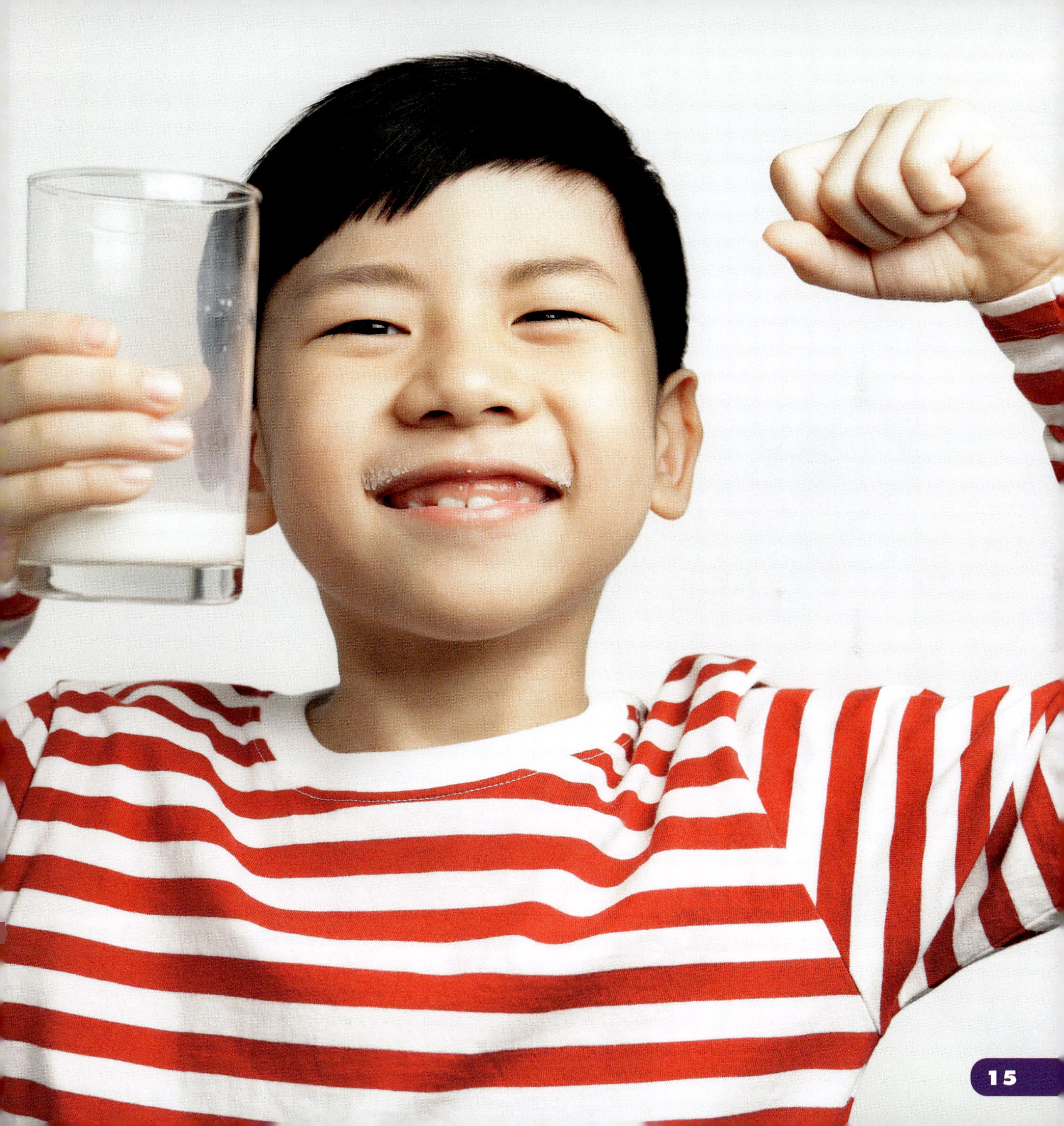

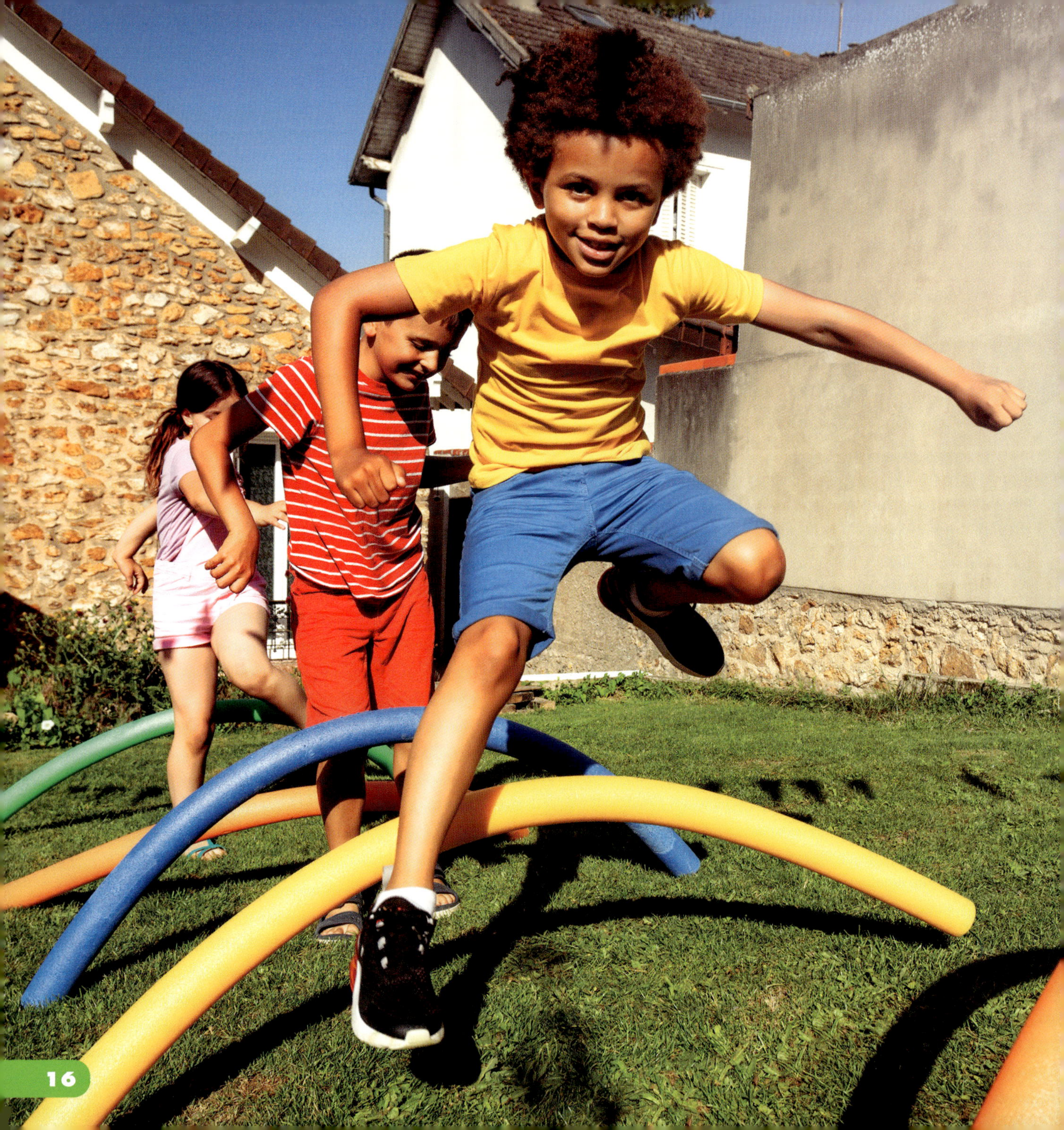

Play for Bones

Jump! Hop! Skip!

Run and play!

Exercise makes bones strong.

Safe Bones

Wear a **helmet** when you ride.

Wear pads to skate.

That keeps bones safe!

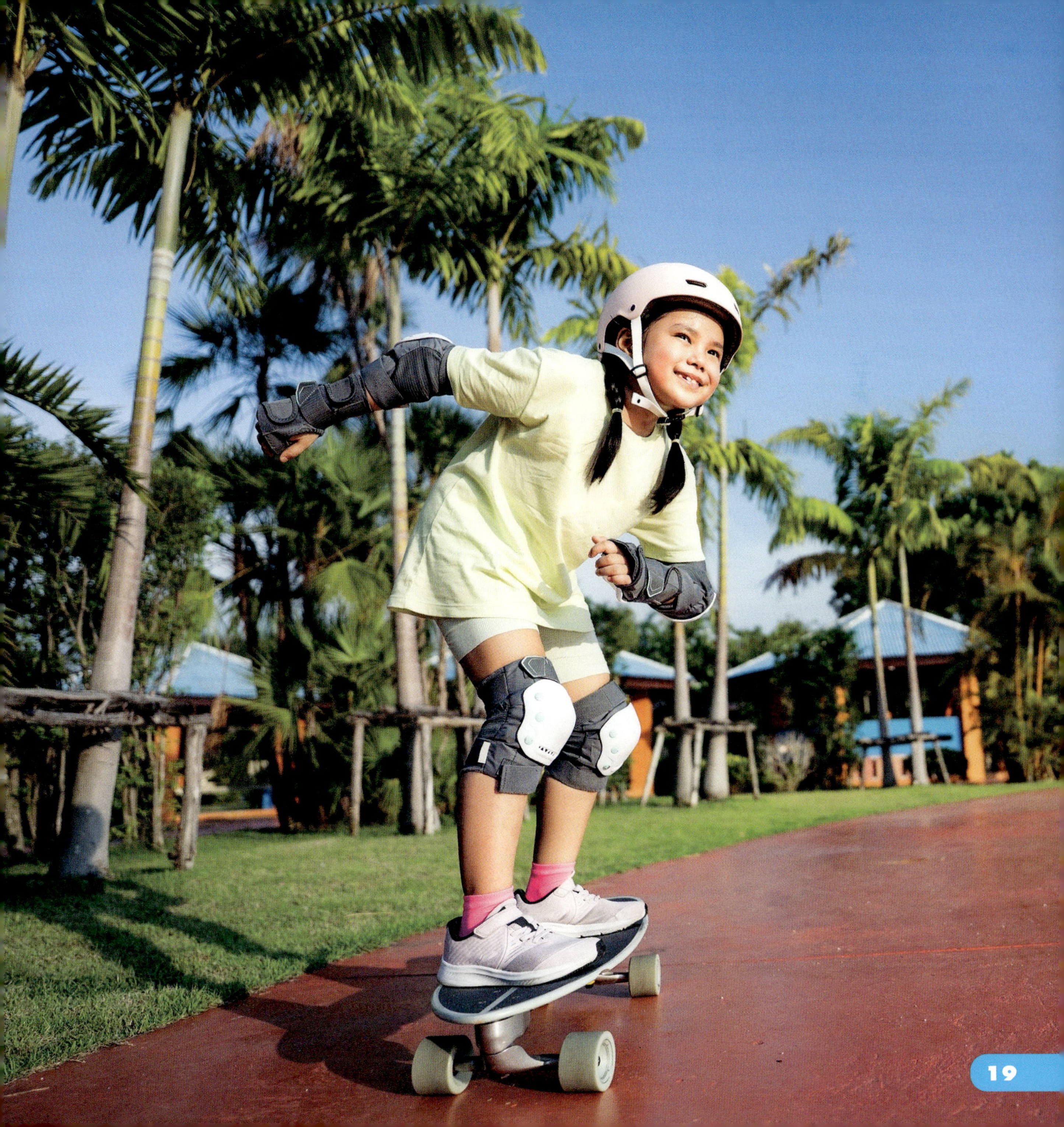

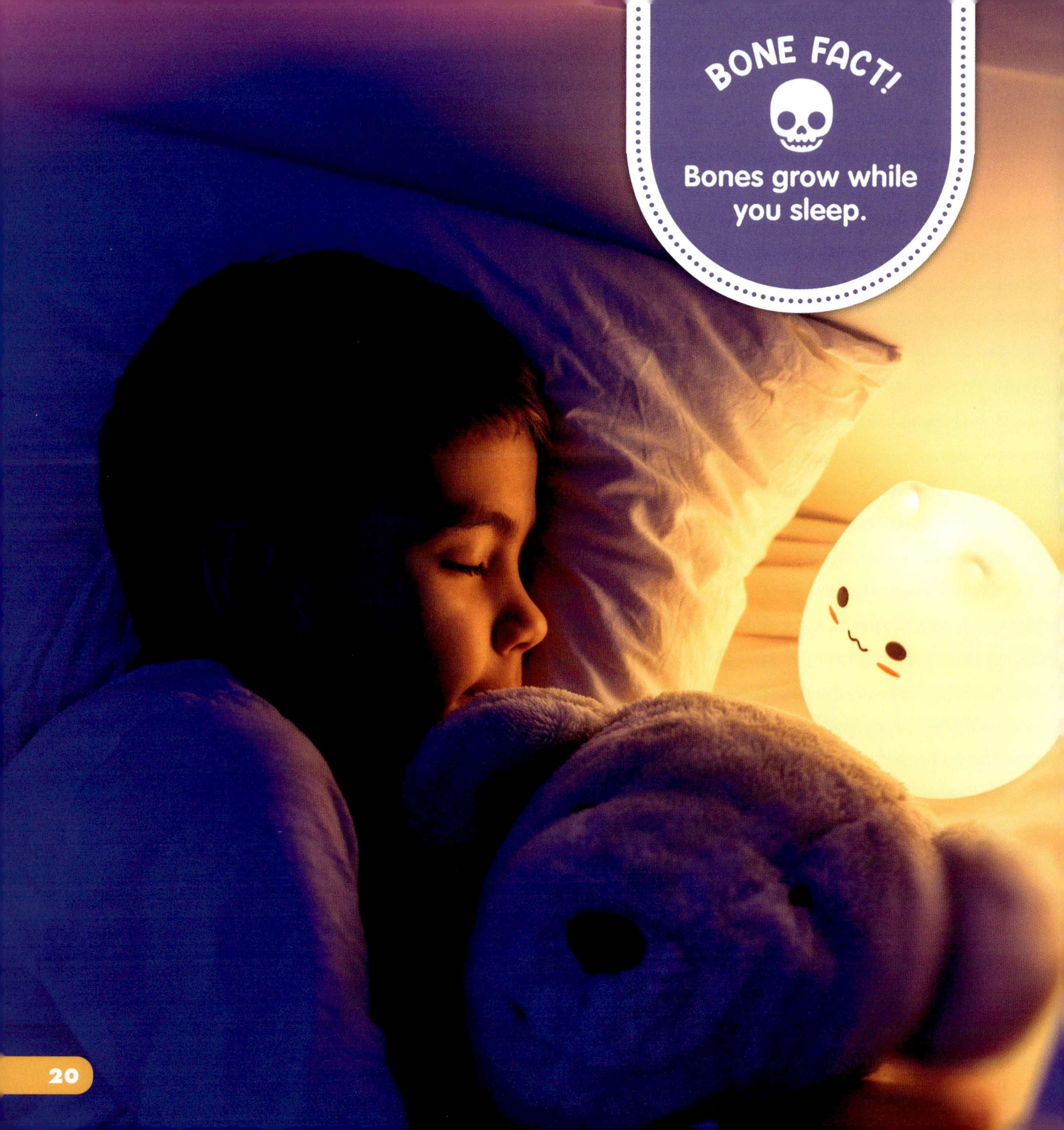

BONE FACT!

Bones grow while you sleep.

Resting Bones

At night, bones rest.

Tomorrow they will help me again.

Glossary

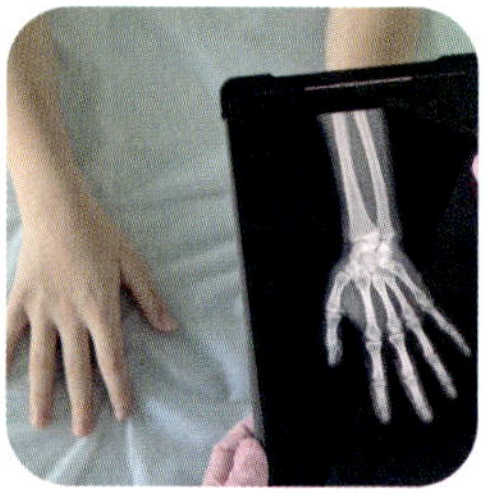

bones (bohnz) hard parts inside your body that help you stand, move, and stay strong

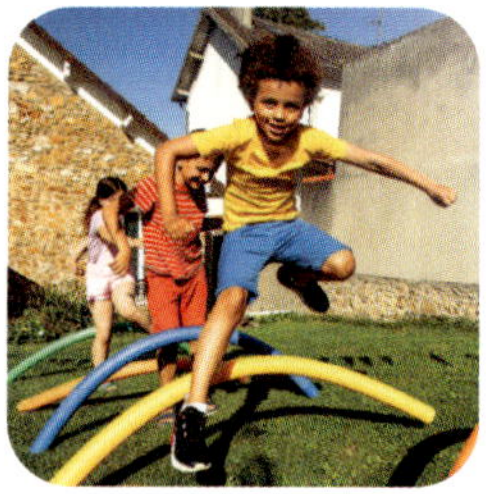

exercise (ek-ser-size) moving your body to play and stay healthy

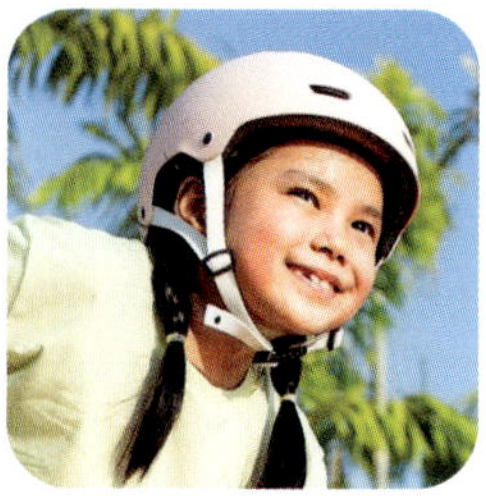

helmet (hel-mit) hard hat that keeps your head safe

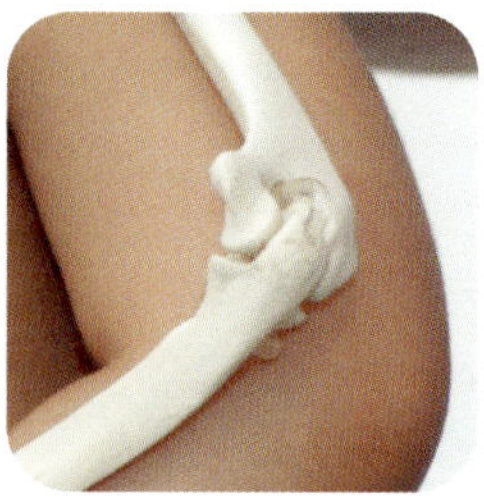

joints (joynts) places where bones meet and bend, like knees and elbows

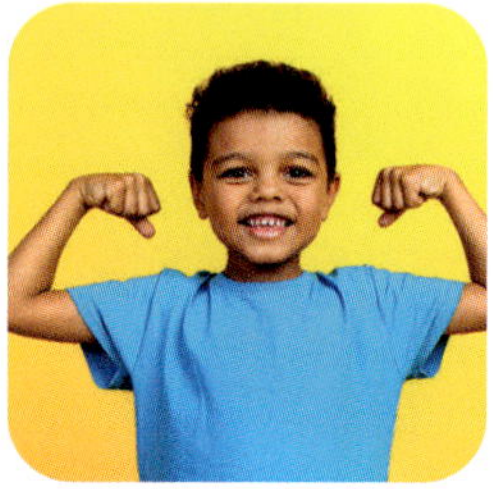

muscles (muh-sulz) soft parts that pull on bones to help you move

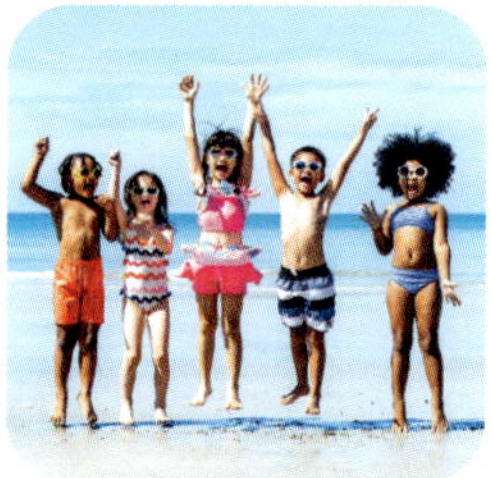

shape (shayp) the way something looks on the outside

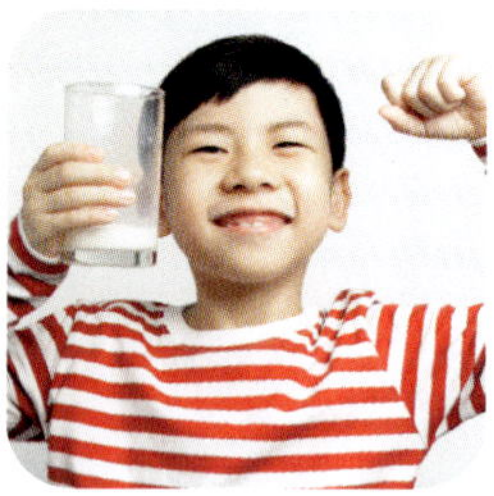

strong (strawng) when something does not break easily

Quiz: My Healthy Bones

1. Do bones help you stand tall?

A. Yes B. No

2. Do joints help your body bend and move?

A. Yes B. No

3. Do helmets help keep bones safe?

A. Yes B. No

4. Do bones grow while you sleep?

A. Yes B. No

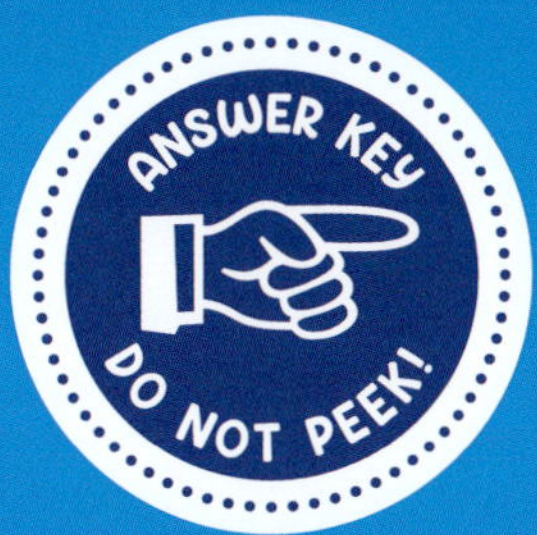

ANSWER KEY:

How many times did you answer yes?

4 Yes: Awesome! You know your bones well.

3 Yes: Great! You learned some new facts.

2 Yes: That's okay! Keep reading.

1 Yes: You're starting to learn. Keep going!

Further Reading

Atkins, Jill. *Bones.* Lerner Publishing, 2024

Rose, Rachel. *My Bones.* Bearport Publishing, 2022

On the Internet

ABCya! Skeletal System Game

https://www.abcya.com/games/skeletal_system

An interactive game where students can label bones or place them in the correct spots on a skeleton.

Dr. Deb's Amazing Skeleton—ABCmouse

https://www.abcmouse.com/learn/game/dr-debs-amazing-skeleton

An interactive game where children can place bones in the correct spots to build a skeleton.

Your Bones (for Kids)—KidsHealth

https://kidshealth.org/en/kids/bones.html

A kid-friendly slideshow explaining how bones work, their functions, and fun facts.

Index

About the Author

Rachel Daniels is a former elementary school teacher who loves reading and discovering new things. She lives in sunny South Florida with her husband, close to her children and grandchildren. When she's not reading or writing, she enjoys playing Canasta with friends. Her goal is to make learning exciting and joyful for young readers everywhere.